L.K. DYL

BULLETPROO

The Ultimate Guide to Effective Dieting, Discover Effective Methods That Can Finally Help You Lose Weight and Keep it Off Starting Today

Descrierea CIP a Bibliotecii Naționale a României
L.K. DYLAN
    BULLETPROOF DIET. The Ultimate Guide to Effective Dieting, Discover Effective Methods That Can Finally Help You Lose Weight and Keep it Off Starting Today / L.K. Dylan. –
Bucharest: Editura My Ebook, 2020
    ISBN 978-606-983-592-0

L.K. DYLAN

BULLETPROOF DIET

The Ultimate Guide to Effective Dieting, Discover Effective Methods That Can Finally Help You Lose Weight and Keep it Off Starting Today

My Ebook Publishing House
Bucharest, 2020

TABLE OF CONTENTS

Introduction 7

Chapter 1: Tracking Your Current Diet 11

Chapter 2. Starting a Food Journal 15

Chapter 3. Getting Ridof Problem Foods 21

Chapter 4. Slow and Steady Wins the Race 28

Chapter 5. Combining Exercise for Best Results 33

Chapter 6. Creating a Calorie Deficit for Weight Loss .. 37

Chapter 7. Introducing Fruits and Vegetables for Weight
   Loss 72

Chapter 8. The Importance of Drinking Water for
   Weight Loss 47

Chapter 9. Lean Meats and Healthy Protein Sources ….. 55

Chapter 10. Planning Meals and Other Tips and Tricks.. 60

Conclusion ……………………………………………. 65

Introduction

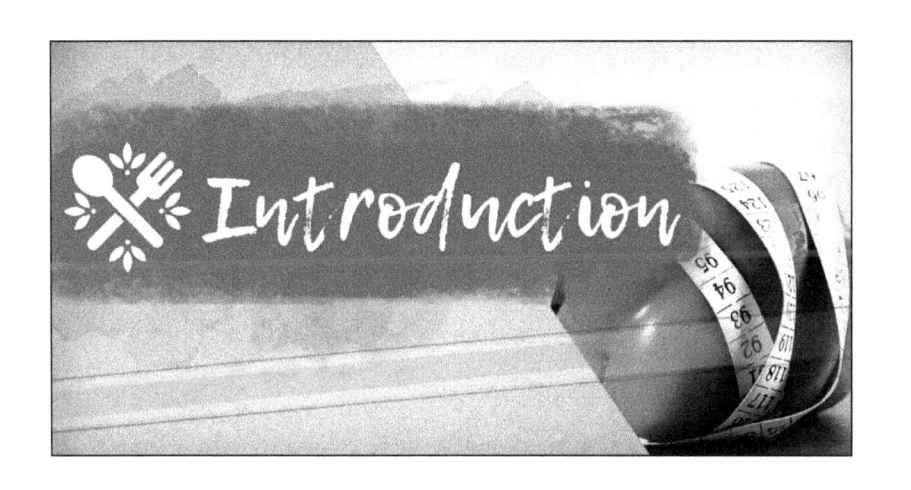

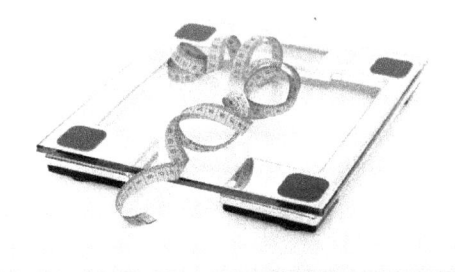

Losing weight is probably one of the things most Americans are concerned with. The obesity epidemic is rampant and can cause a lot of people to have many health issues and other difficulties. Weight loss has become more and more important, not just as a beauty standard or trend, but because it can be sodangerous to live your life on processed foods.

Processed foods are probably one of the leading killers of people who suffer from obesity in North America.

There are so many dangers to processed foods. For example, they are full of hidden fats and sugars. The ingredients and processed foods are highly unnatural. They can contribute to several health problems, including hypertension and diabetes. If you try to go through the shelves in a grocery store and avoid high fructose corn syrup, but you'll probably find that it is nearly impossible. High fructose corn syrup is very unhealthy could be considered just another way of saying pure sugar. Except, this type of sugar is more difficult for you to get rid of in your body.

Everybody is looking for a miracle cure when it comes to weight loss. It can be very easy to gain weight and very difficult to get rid of it once it's there. When this is the case, it can become almost impossible, or so it feels, to get back to the state of being that you want to be in. Our bodies can be viewed as instruments that's are molded and shaped by our habits and behaviors. For any diet to work, you have to first change yourself and your outlook. Only then will you be able to stay consistent with the effort that makes it possible to actually lose weight and stay on the proper diet plan.

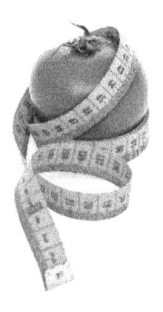

Becoming malnourished is actually very simple, whether you are being fed every day or not. When we eat, the foods that sustain us are usually junk foods, and they will keep us alive. At least in the short term. However, in the long term, it will shorten your lifespan because you are not eating foods that are nourishing to your body. Without the proper vitamins and minerals, you will ultimately find that you are sluggish and weak, and have a difficult time concentrating. That's because you are not being nourished, and nutritional deficiencies can cause a whole slew of health problems that are highly dangerous and can ultimately interfere with your quality of life.

So how can you possibly begin to lose weight and provide yourself with this sustenance that you need to thrive, rather than simply float on by in your life? By following the guidelines of the Foolproof diet, you will ultimately find that you are taking the steps that need to be taken in order to develop a healthy lifestyle that will provide you with the energy you need in order to continue to burn calories and make weight loss a success. Even if you aren't simply trying to lose weight and just want to create a better lifestyle for yourself, the Foolproof diet will give you all the information that you need in order to begin changing your life, starting right now.

Chapter 1

Tracking Your Current Diet

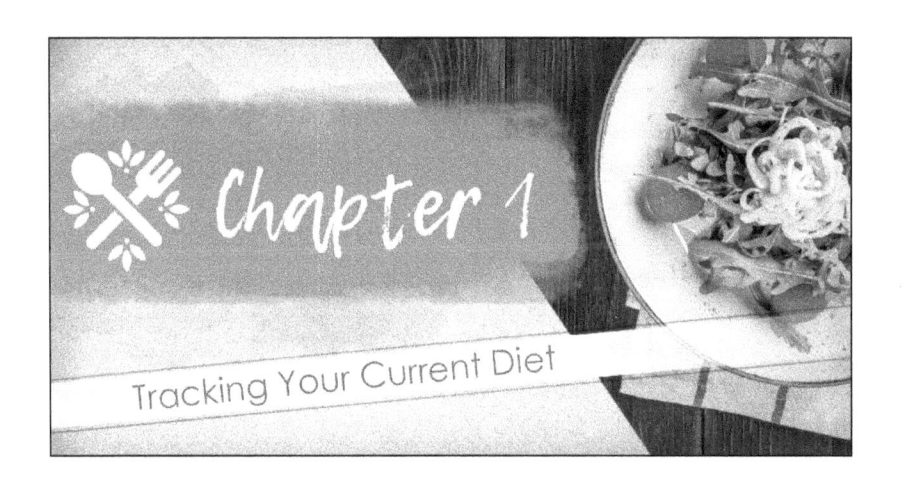

They say that the definition of insanity is doing the same thing over and over and expecting different results. That is never more true than it is when it comes to weight loss. To become well on your way toward achieving your goals, you first must know yourself and understand your habits. How and what you eat can change everything when it comes to your efforts to lose weight, and if you aren't willing to track your diet and see the ways it needs to change, then unfortunately you may never meet your weight loss goals or potential.

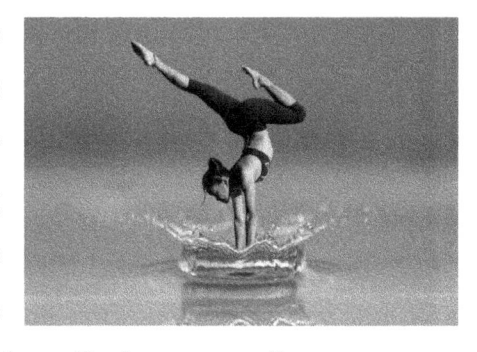

One of the greatest ways that you can begin to embark upon a foolproof diet is in tracking the diet that you are currently on. What do you beat every day? What is the basic outline of what you eat? Are you doing your best to take care of your body, or do you give yourself way too much leeway? Are you tired and busy and feel like you have no other option than to eat fast food all the time? Or do you simply not have a clue in the kitchen and have found yourself feeling frustrated by the time and preparation it can take to prepare a healthy meal at the end of a long day?

Whatever the case may be, tracking your current diet is a great way for you to begin changing your life. But how do you begin to track your current diet? First of all, you should have a notebook or journal where you enter in what you have been every day. Start with the beginning, and if you have a difficult time drinking water as opposed to other sugary and unhealthy drinks, then you should also include what you have consumed of water as well. Start from the time you wake up and don't stop until you have finished eating for the day. If you get up to snack, either include these instances after they have happened for the next day if you feel too tired. However, the best results, when you are completely transparent about your dietary habits and you record them immediately.

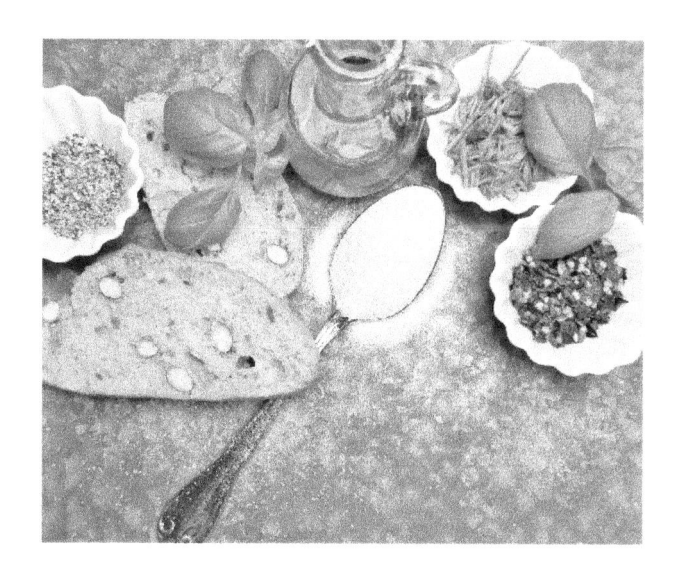

Tracking your diet is easier than it sounds. What can be difficult is reading through the entries and realizing that you haven't been doing what is best for your body and mind. When that is the case you may begin to feel like you are failing at your goals and it can give you a sense of shame and low self-esteem that can make it difficult to keep moving forward toward achieving your goal.

But rather than beating yourself up about it, you should view it as an opportunity to do better for yourself in the future. For most people, it can take a while to develop a habit. In fact, biologically it can be 7 days before a habit is formed by repeating positive behaviors. When those new habits are reinforced you would be surprised by just how hard to recognize yourself. Instead of living life consumed by the effects of your negative habits and bad patterns, you may discover that you are a strong person who is capable of making great changes for yourself and your environment.

To begin such a venture, you should definitely begin by tracking the current diet that you are following, even if it turns out that your current habits are not very healthy.

Everybody makes mistakes, and when you follow a bad habit long enough, it can be difficult to do any differently. However, the trick is not in shaming yourself but in accepting where you are at and being completely honest and transparent about it. Not everybody is able to view the hard truths of a situation with the strength it takes to implement changes using the information they have observed about themselves, but it is something that can be drastically healing and a very useful tool in making positive life changes, now and for the future days to come.

Chapter 2
Starting a Food Journal

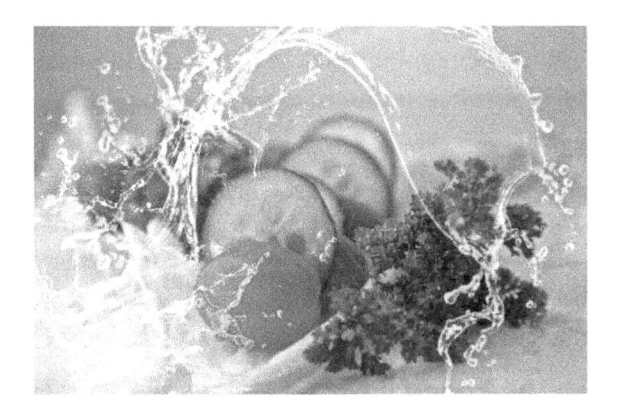

Once you have begun to track your current diet and have a good understanding of what it is that you are doing that may prevent you from making progress on your weight loss journey, it is a good idea to begin a food journal. A food journal is a great way to help you to keep track of recipes you want to prepare and creating meal plans that will help you to stick to a healthy diet full of fruits and vegetables. Not only that but it will help you a lot in creating the type of accountability you need to make healthy changes and stick with them.

Your food journal can consist of the same record you took to see what your every day diet is generally like. But it doesn't have to be. You could also use a different notebook to create your food journal. The food journal is a very useful tool in aiding weight loss and keeping on track with your diet. You want something that will help you to take accountability for what you are putting into your body every day, otherwise it can be difficult to remember that we are staying on track for a reason.

Humans have a tendency to think on a short-term scale and lack the ability to plan for the future. When you are able to plan for future, such as using a food journal to help you to list ingredients and meals you need or would like to try, it can really give you a solid foundation and give you a rare opportunity to see how every single tiny choice you make can be something that either improves your future or prevents you from becoming the person that you want to be.

When you understand the profound consequences of your every action, it will help you to think more in depth about the choices that you have to make on a daily basis. When you don't understand, it can be nearly impossible to stay on track with a program or regimen that provides your body with the healing sustenance that it requires in order to thrive.

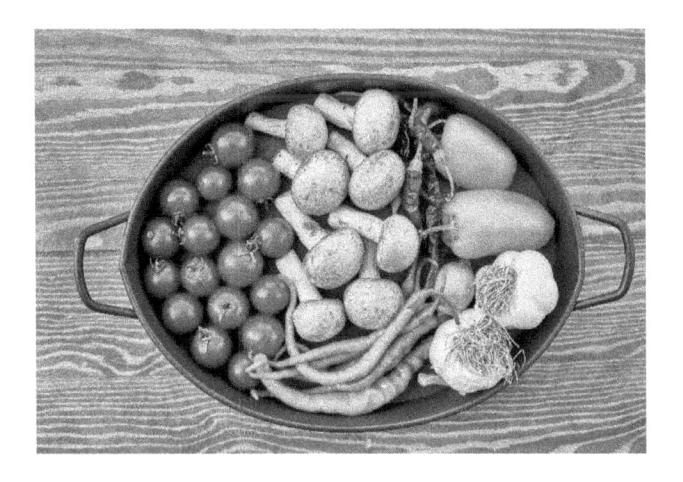

It can be so easy to be addicted to bad foods. But by utilizing a food journal, you will be able to see when and where your cravings for certain foods may creep up. For example, you may realize that when you are stressed out or too tired to cook, you begin to crave things that are far more unhealthy for you. But when you are less stressed out or have plenty of time to cook, you find that you are a lot more okay with taking the extra effort to make sure you are eating healthy foods and doing things that will move your health forward.

To best utilize a food journal, you should first and foremost make sure that you are being honest with your entries. Write in it every day, and try to record the foods you are eating directly after eating them. If you want to, you could also make a record of their nutritional value so you have a sense of what you are consuming on any given day, that way you aren't surprised at the end of the week if you find you have either gained or lost weight.

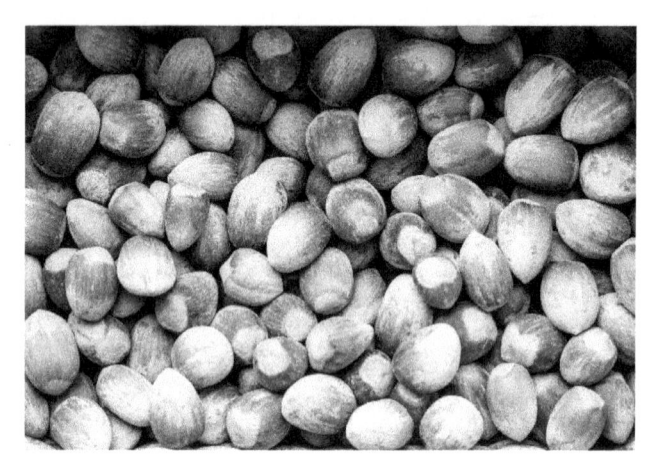

Next, as you may have considered with the word "journal" involved, you should also record how you felt about the foods you were eating and how you were feeling prior to eating said foods. You should also take some time to consider how you felt *after* eating these foods, because it can be very telling of a food's nutritional content and compatibility with your body if you are able to accurately assess the moods you have following a certain food. For example, if you find you are intolerant to nuts or soy, but don't have an outright allergy, you may find that after consuming such things you feel more irritable or moody or agitated. This is because your body has sensed a threat and you are receiving a stress response in order to deal with the body's perceived threat. Pay close attention to what works with your body and what probably doesn't agree. That will give you a chance to really assess what foods work for you in a way that is personal and in depth. This way, you will truly understand why it is not good for you to eat certain things, while others may not be so difficult for you to enjoy.

Overall, having a food journal is a good way to get in touch with yourself and with your food. In most cultures, food is a spiritual experience that should be shared and enjoyed. It is given far more consideration than it is generally in north America. For this reason, it can be a great and healing thing to be able to take comfort in specific foods knowing exactly what type of relationships our bodies will have with those foods when they are put into our bodies.

One of the most important keys in creating a foolproof diet plan is in knowing our bodies and being in touch with ourselves enough that we are making good choices as often as possible. when we are out of synch with ourselves, it can become nearly impossible to do what is best for us. But having a food journal is a great way to help us get our bodies and minds connected and focused on one of the key elements of improving our health and wellbeing.

Chapter 3

Getting Rid of Problem Foods

We all have our vices, and these problem foods can sometimes be the downfall of any well-intentioned dieter. Trying to maintain her self control can be very difficult if we aren't careful. This is especially true of dietary habits, because most of the time we develop them because we want an easy solution to a ravenous hunger. When we don't find that solution in an easy way, we get agitated and frustrated, and often times give up entirely on cooking. Have you ever had one of those days where you can find something easy to make it home and so you went out and bought something easy instead?

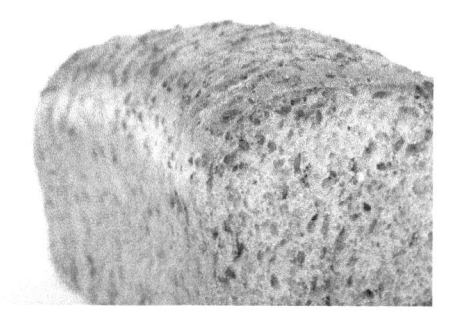

Now is the time to begin identifying these behaviors and seeing how they are affecting you in the long term. Sometimes it can be very dangerous to have a reliance on fast and easy foods. Processed foods come with a whole slew of potential health problems that can make your body suffer over the course of time, even if it feels like a quick solution and you feel good because of all of the fats and sugars that are giving your body chemical reactions that convince you that you are enjoying this food and that is what your body wants or needs.

Problem foods are in every house, and every cupboard or pantry may have problem foods lurking there waiting to be discovered. If you find that you are fighting off the urge to eat problem foods that you have in your own home, then that is the first sign that you should get rid of them.

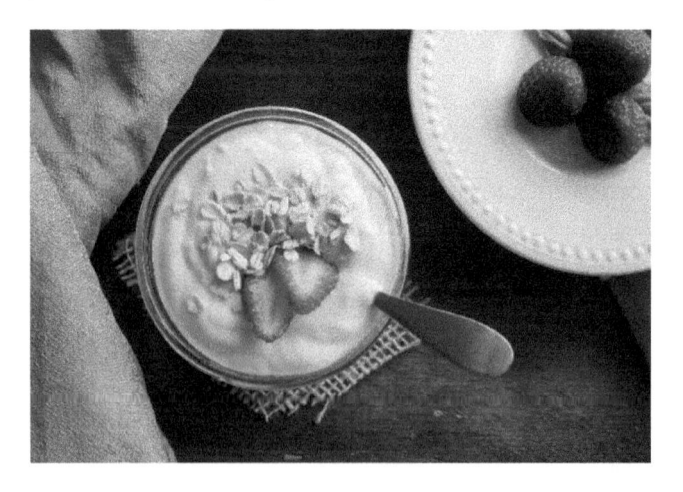

First of all, you are going to want to get rid of sodas and other sugary drinks. Most people don't realize just how much sugar is in juice. We think that it is healthy because it comes from fruit, but fruit is full of natural sugars, and when it is juiced, we are not getting the natural fibers that actually make the fruit healthy. Instead, we are getting a concoction of concentrated sugars from the fruits that are present in the juice and added sugars as well most of the time. This is true of other foods that have been deemed healthy, such as yogurt or granola bars. They are packed full of sugar, and in eating those sugars, it can be almost impossible to lose weight and see any results.

If you want to get rid of sugar entirely, you probably could, and you would see very fast results from that as well. For the most part, at least try to make sure that you are limiting your sugar intake to about 30 g of sugar per day. This can be difficult, because when you start to look at the ingredients list on your foods and your soft drinks, you find that most of these drinks have two servings in them, and a single serving is about maximum the sugar that you should be intaking if you want to see results in the weight loss department.

Don't be upset at yourself for having been tricked by these supposedly healthy foods. Just remember the next time that you are shopping not to invest in them. They are only going to hold you back from achieving your goals, and this can have a very negative effect on your self-esteem. Keep after grocery list, and if you see them in your house, you can either give them away or throw them away. Something many people struggle with is a sense of feeling as if they are obligated to eat the food that is in front of them. This can be theresult of childhood conditioning by parents who wanted to make sure that we were well fed whether we like the food in front of us or not.

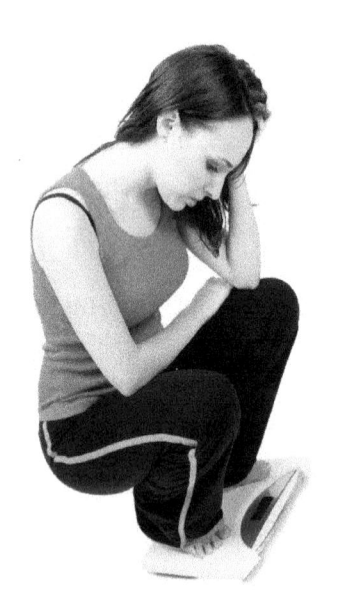

Try not to feel bad for wasting food that is going to contribute to either weight gain or potential health problems in the future. If you know that it is something that isn't good for you, but you have a lot of it, see what you can donate to a food bank or give away to friends or other family members who are not on the same weight loss or health journey that you are on. Sometimes, this is the only way to make great changes. We have to be stronger than our negative impulses, and the only way to begin to do that is to try.

However, don't do it in a rapid-fire session that is too fast and extreme for you. Instead, consult chapter 4 of the ways that you can begin to implement positive changes in a way that is not overwhelming. When we are overwhelmed, they can be almost impossible for positive changes that we attempt to make to stick with us. We can become consumed by the stress of doing new things that are unfamiliar and difficult. For this reason, make sure that you are following the guidelines expressed in the next chapter so that you are able to get rid of the unhealthy foods that are preventing you from living the lifestyle that you dream of.

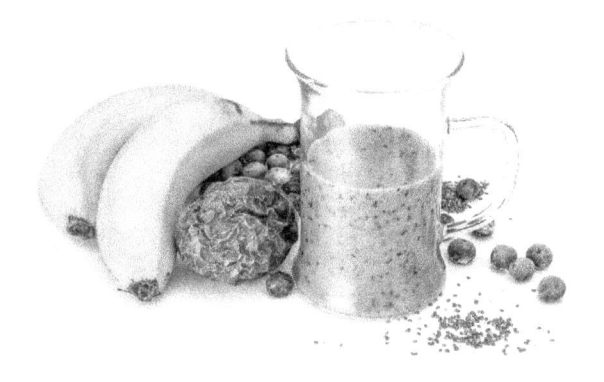

Instead, take stock of the unhealthy foods that are making regular appearances in your life and make an active effort to cut them out. Whether that is by getting rid of the ones that you already have or by avoiding buying them in the first place, you are going to be on the right track in avoiding these foods.

Some examples of foods you may want to avoid are the following:
- Processed foods
- Candy
- Foods high in sugar
- Foods high in fat
- Foods high in sodium
- Soft drinks
- Juices
- Smoothies that consist of more than 2 parts fruit 3 parts vegetable
- Starches and starchy foods like potatoes and white flour products (pasta noodles, etc.)

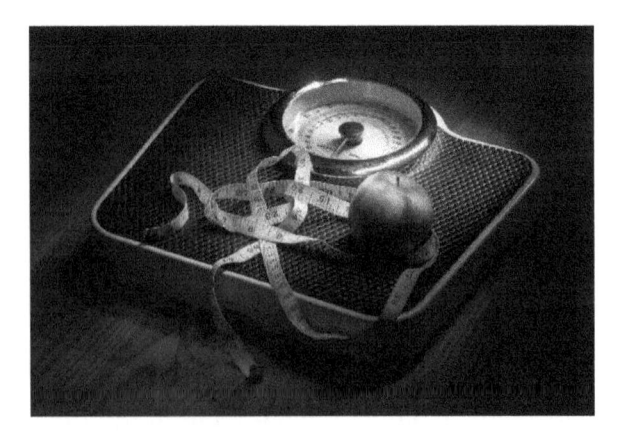

Use your common sense and do whatever is possible for you to avoid the foods you know are going to be problematic and hinder your weight loss journey. Without your own discretion, it is going to be difficult. You have to know what affects your body and how, and generally speaking, it can be very difficult for our bodies to handle an overload of sugars and fats, especially those present in the easy to access foods in North American culture, such as fast food and processed, boxed foods.

Most of us instinctively know the foods that are bad for us when we see them. It is usually an exercise in self-control to be making good use of the foods that we know are good for us and turning down the ones that are quick and easy. If you pre-prepare your healthy meals, they too can become quick and easy for you. It is all a matter of perspective. If you re-train your brain to believe that you are making the best possible choice for yourself, getting rid of problematic foods should not be an issue for you at all.

Chapter 4

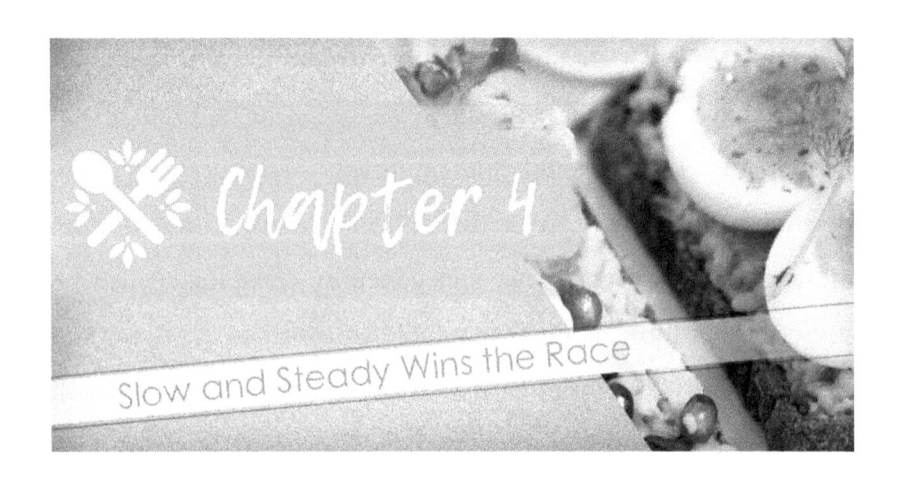

Slow and Steady Wins the Race

It can be harder than many people realize to begin a new healthy habit, but when you are dedicated to achieving your goals, then there is nothing that should stop you and get in your way. However, a lot of what prevents us from reaching goals is a mental block that can create many disturbances and disruptions in our lives. Fortunately for us, there are ways that we can begin to care for our bodies and minds and prepare ourselves mentally for the strenuous task ahead of us.

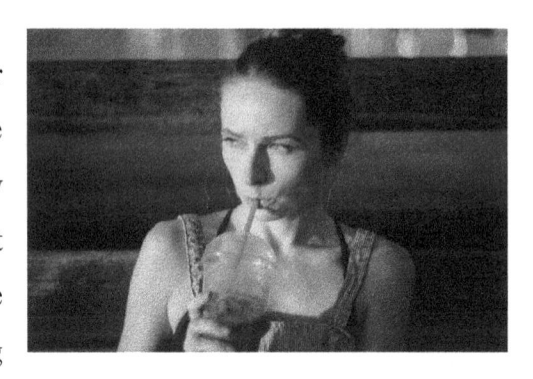

One great way to help us get ahead before we even begin is to have realistic expectations. Don't eat a healthy meal one day a week and expect for it to be enough to lose weight. In fact, that is far from the truth. In order to lose weight, you have to make sure that you are doing everything in your power to follow through on goals, even when you relapse.

It is harder for us to achieve goals when we are not being realistic. To begin formulating a new habit, we need to start slow. Introduce it gradually, in small steps and steady doses, rather than imposing unrealistic expectations on yourself that will be nearly impossible to work toward and maintain. Instead of making several drastic lifestyle changes at once, instead, do your best to implement small changes and do them gradually until they feel like a normal part of your life.

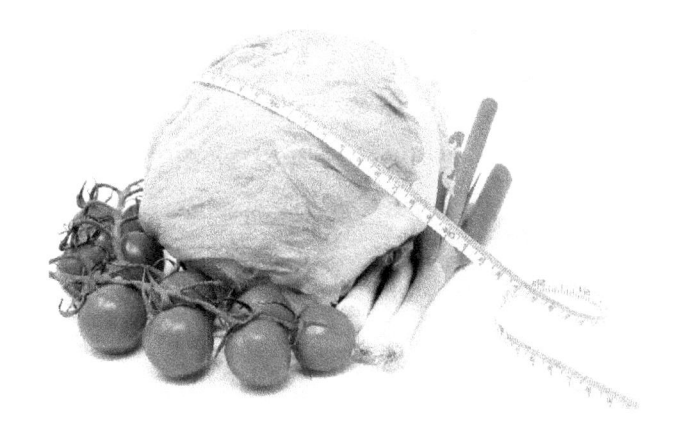

We have to start small. If we take on too much, it is the surest way to failure. Integrating new habits into our lives should be done carefully. Start with small steps to begin with. For example, instead of putting out every single unhealthy food that you are addicted to it one, try starting out with cutting out one thing at a time. Go for about a week of cutting out that food before cutting out another food that you know you should get rid of.

Although this process may seem slow, it is a sure fire way to make sure that the changes you are trying to implement will last. Instead of overloading your mind with a lot of different stressful changes, it is very helpful to be able to take a step back and allow your body the time to get use to making healthier choices.

It can be physically stressful to make changes in your diet, so try to go easy on yourself. Relapses can and probably will happen, but what you have to remember is that you are doing this to get healthy, and not to punish yourself. If you make a mistake, so be it. But leave your mistakes in the past and continue trying to move forward. Don't let one mistake become a slippery slope back into your unhealthy lifestyle. Although it may seem difficult at first, you will be surprised by just how easy it is to begin to get use to the lifestyle of making healthy, body conscious choices that will reward you and pave the way toward a healthier future for yourself.

Don't overdo it. You need to make sure that you are taking on your challenges in a way that will provide you with the resources you need at your disposal to thrive. When you are not able to do so, that is when things get difficult. You could try to set aside a date bi-weekly to begin to introduce new habits and eating changes so that you can begin to take on all the new habits that you want to develop in order to make your lifestyle the healthiest it can possibly be.

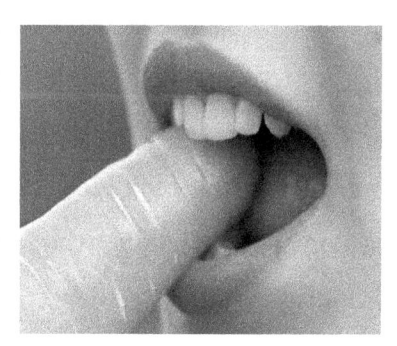

And this isn't true of just changing your diet and precluding unhealthy foods from your lifestyle. This can work for just about any lifestyle choice you could possibly make. If you wanted to begin learning a new language for example, you could begin slow by starting a new regimen of, once every week, studying that language. You could eventually bring the number of days you practice your language up until you are practicing two to three times a week, or even setting time aside daily for that venture. As long as you start off slow, you will ultimately be able to develop a habit so that you are heading closer and closer toward the life you have always dreamed of for yourself.

It is more than possible for you to achieve your goals. You just have to approach them with realistic expectations of yourself and the biological reality that it takes a long time to develop specific habits, while others can sometimes come more naturally. Either way, don't overload your brain by trying to make huge changes all at once. A gradual ability to take in the changes will provide you with the structure you need to make long-lasting choices that will improve your life from here on out.

Chapter 5
Combining Exercise for Best Results

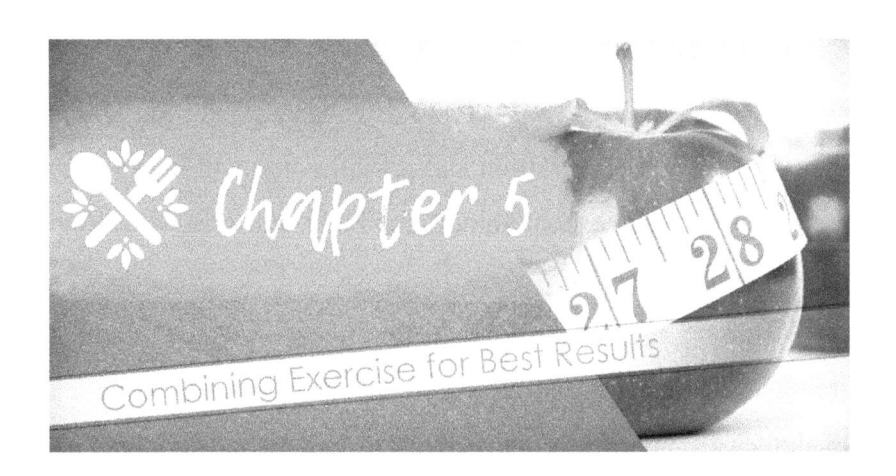

A healthy diet is an incredible thing to have, but if your goal is weight loss, any diet that is healthy and nutritious is best paired with an exercise routine that suits your lifestyle and provides you with all of the calorie-burning opportunities you can get! When you lose weight, it means you are creating a deficit in calories. This will be discussed further in the next chapter.

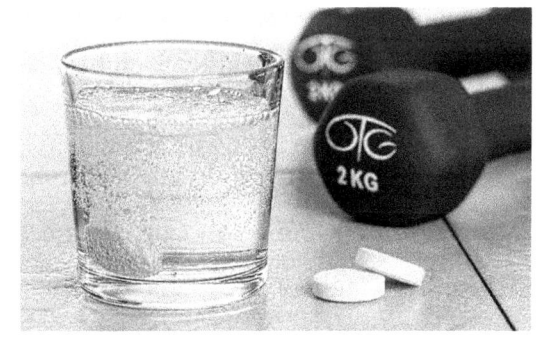

In summary, you want to burn more calories than you consume, and to do so you need to establish a good routine that includes both proper nutrition and activities that will help you to burn fat away while nourishing your body, muscles, and mind all at the same time.

Burning calories can be difficult, especially if you are living a stagnant lifestyle. When you are stuck working behind a computer all day, it can get difficult to move your body and do the exercise that you need to do in order to keep your blood flowing properly every day. That makes it even harder to burn calories and stay at a healthy weight, let alone lose excess fat that is being stored in our bodies.

When we are living a sedentary lifestyle, it is incredibly bad for our bodies. We can't just go on a diet and expect fast and healthy weight loss results without considering what we need to do physically in order to contribute to a sure-fire and foolproof way of losing weight. If weight loss isn't your goal, that is fine. However, it is still important to maintain a regular exercise routine so that you are not harming yourself. Lack of exercise makes it difficult to get rid of toxins in the body, especially those that are stored inside our body fat. This can make it close to impossible to lose weight. Toxins tend to get bound to our fat cells and the combination makes it difficult to get rid of the excess body fat inside of us.

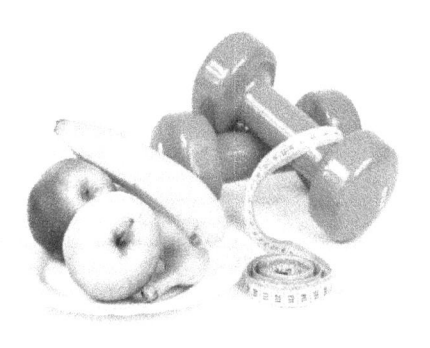

That's why it is so important to exercise. Not only do we begin to sweat out the toxins and other bad things in our bodies, but we can also begin to build muscle. When we build muscle, it helps us to burn fat all throughout the day. In fact, strength training is a great way to build the muscles that we need in order to maintain a healthy metabolism so that we are able to thrive. When we are building muscles, they provide the body with a constant ability to burn the fuel that we provide to them. When we are burning more fuel than we are consuming, that is when we begin to lose fat and really make a difference in our weight loss journeys.

It can also be very beneficial to include cardio exercises as well. It is hard for the body to lose weight if you are not engaging in activities that make you sweat and keep your heart rate up. Cardio is a way to burn a lot of calories and improve the deficit of calories consumed versus calories burned. That means that you will be losing weight. This is especially true if you are making intelligent and health conscious food choices throughout the day rather than eating foods that are bad for you and causing you to gain weight or hold on to stubborn fat rather than releasing it through exercise and smart eating.

You can probably lose weight without exercising, but the results will be minimal at best. In order to undertake a foolproof diet plan, moving your body and getting the blood pumping will be an indisputable way for you to lose weight and get yourself on track toward achieving the body you have always wanted. Because being the best version of yourself is something that you deserve, and exercising will help you to do that.

Chapter 6

Creating a Calorie Deficit for Weight Loss

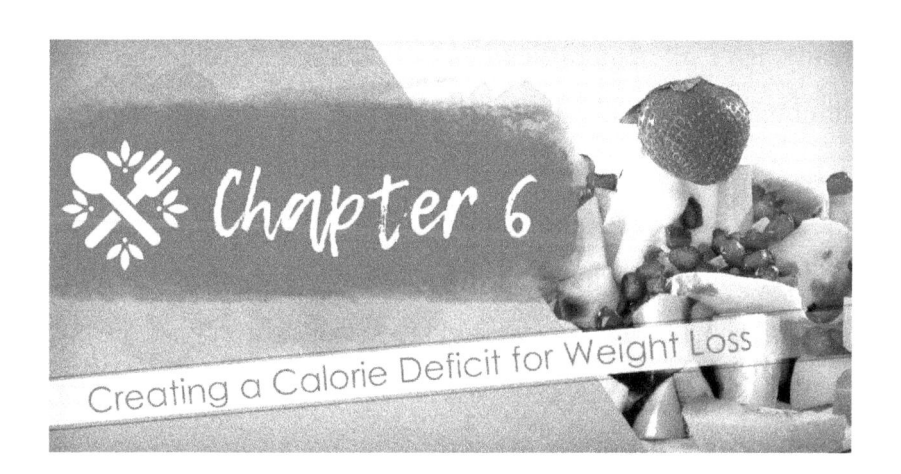

Most people dread the idea of counting calories, and they probably should. It is boring, abysmal, and can create an unhealthy fixation on your body image and the foods you are willing to consume. It can be a very limiting way to live your life.

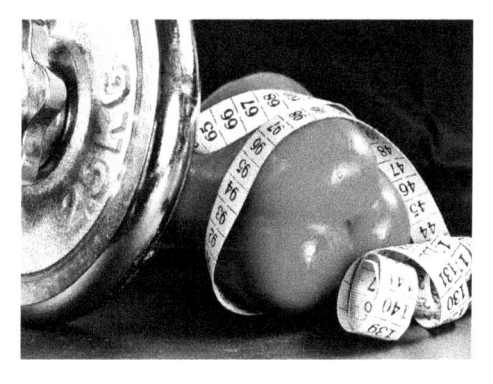

However, by following the foolproof diet plan and eating a vegetable and protein based diet while coupling it with muscle-building exercises that make it possible to burn through your fat in no time at all, you will find that creating a calorie deficit really isn't all that difficult, and it doesn't have to be very limiting in the foods that you eat at all!

As long as you are eating foods that are building your body up rather than making it more difficult for you to sustain yourself and maintain a healthy lifestyle, creating a calorie deficit with the healthy food choices that are outlined in this book is simple. It is a good way to ensure a foolproof diet that won't end up backfiring on you.

Every pound of fat consists of about 3,500 calories. In order to lose a pound of fat, you need to be able to burn about that many calories; not counting what you consume per day. At this point, it would generally make a difference to cut out about 500 calories per day in order to lose a pound of fat per week.

Remember, it is better to do things right than it is to do them quickly. You don't want to be trying to rush yourself into rapid weight loss. Doing so can have adverse results on your health and your physical body. Losing weight too quickly can actually result in loose or sagging skin. You want to do things naturally, even if it is slower than the easy 100 pound weight loss that the latest trend diet is promising within the next week. Losing weight that quickly is vastly unhealthy.

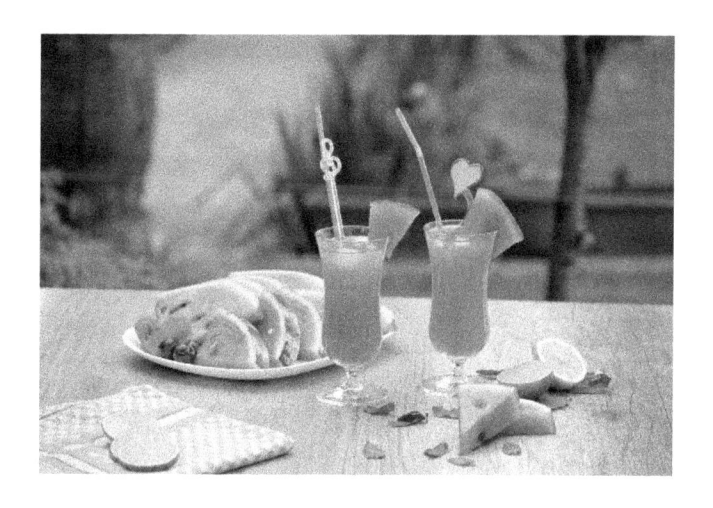

A fairly healthy calorie deficit would be to cut 500 calories or less out of your diet every day. So, taking what you are eating typically into consideration, you either need to cut down on that many calories when eating, or exercise and create a deficit that way. Of course, as mentioned previously, combining a healthy diet and exercise is the fastest path to foolproof weight loss.

No diet plan is perfect, and most of us are well aware of that fact. In fact, many fad diets are incredibly unhealthy and unsafe. Some of them can even have life-long health consequences. This is something that can be very difficult to deal with without adequate attention paid to the potential side effects of the diets that you are trying out. The safest and most effective way to lose weight is by following a healthy eating plan and maintaining regular exercise.

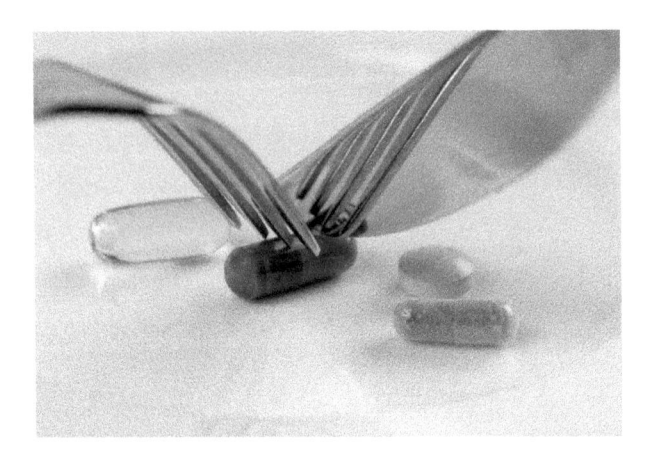

Other diets, such as the hcg diet or others that may promote unhealthy actions or taking pills that are not necessarily tried and true, can be devastating to your body over the long term. Instead of being swayed by the promise of rapid weight loss, try to picture all the things that will come with it. Saggy skin and a whole slew of health problems that will make losing weight the least of your worries. It doesn't sound worth it, does it? That's because it isn't.

Remembering to count your calories is something that seems to be compulsive and sometimes can become an unhealthy obsession, so do your best to remember that you are doing this for your health, not because you want to look a certain way. Making sure you are pursuing a lifestyle change for the right reasons is one of the most crucial ways of ensuring that you are able to make the lasting changes that you need.

Pay close attention to your calorie intake, but not so much that it becomes an obsession. If you are worried you have eaten more calories than you burned in a day, simply go for a walk or a jog and let yourself try to relax. As long as you are making a consistent effort and don't give up, you will achieve your goals. What matters most is continuing to make progress and never letting yourself get so discouraged that you end up halting all of your efforts entirely.

The trick in losing weight is to create a calorie deficit, and that's exactly what you are going to do if you are reliably counting your calories and making an effort to eat nourishing foods and pair a good diet with regular exercise. It may help you to visit with a nutritionist so they can help you to take your individual needs into consideration as you begin this new journey in your life. That way, every step of the way is done with efficiency and care, and you are giving yourself and your health the royal treatment that it deserves!

Chapter 7

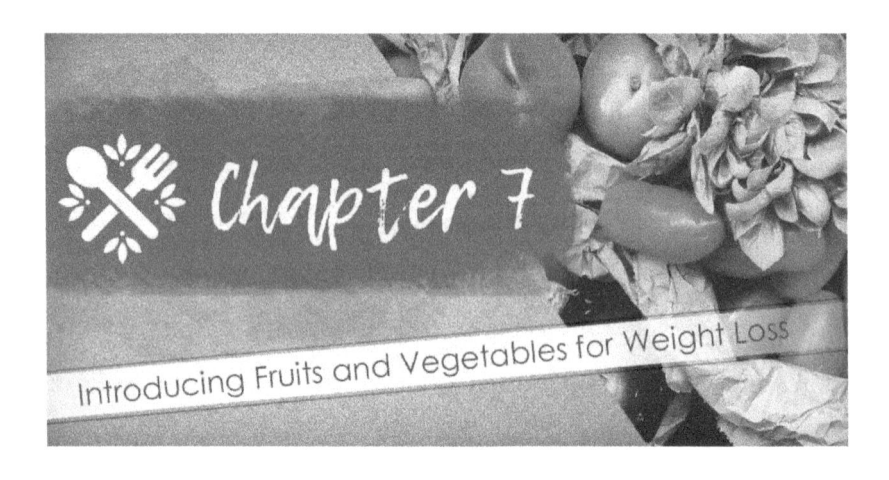

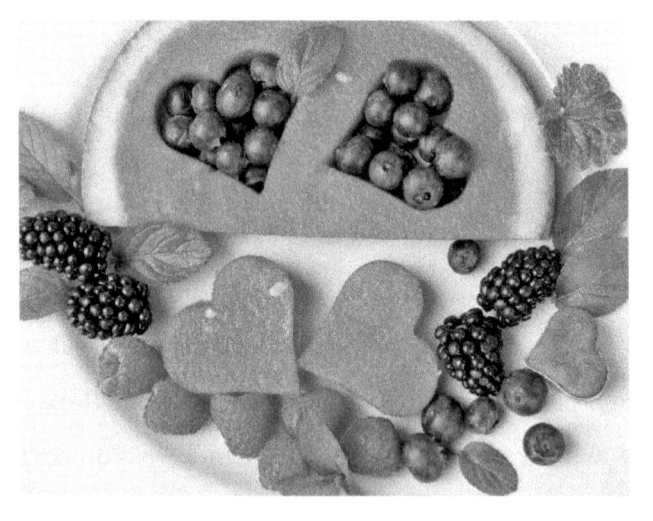

Introducing Fruits and Vegetables for Weight Loss

One thing that is drastically lacking in the typical standard American diet is healthy and natural foods. Fruits and vegetables are often bypassed for easy to access canned goods that are usually strung out versions of their former nutritionally packed selves. It can be a very dangerous thing to become reliant on processed and canned foods. They are full of hidden sugars and fats and can easily pack on the pounds and leave your body starved of nutrients if you aren't careful.

What many people who are consumed with losing weight don't seem to realize is that fruits and vegetables are actually very helpful in this arena. Not only do they stave away hunger pangs, but they are rich in water content and fibers that help you to digest your foods and get rid of excessive waste in your body. Not only that, but because of those fibers, you may find that you get filled up faster. And generally speaking there is not much of a limit to how many fruits and vegetables you should eat in a day. They make great snacks for hungry dieters, assuming you are not diabetic or have some other condition that may make it necessary to avoid natural sugars.

Fruits and vegetables are great for jump starting the metabolism and creating a great snack that is low in calories and high in water content and fiber. This means that you can generally eat as many vegetables as you want to without having to worry excessively about gaining weight. This is actually great news, because instead of starving yourself, you can eat an abundance of nourishing foods that provide you with a great amount of sustenance. Healthy eating will help to provide you with the energy you need to embark upon the other great aspects of weight loss, such as being active and maintaining a regular exercise routine.

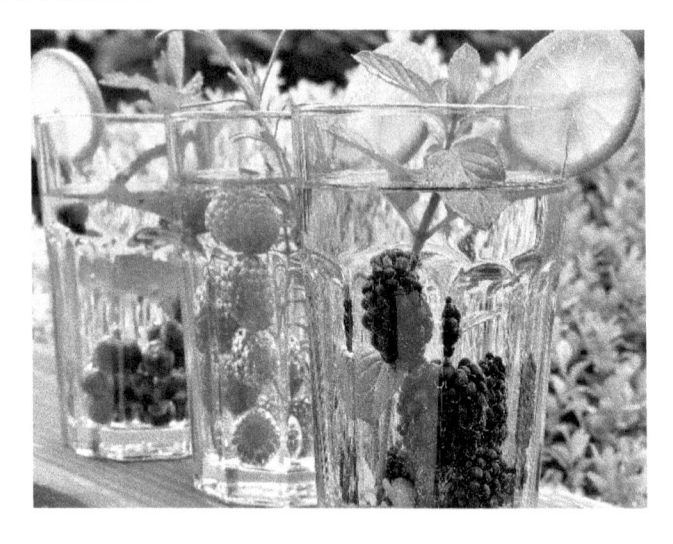

It will also help you to stay mentally alert, which can be a great thing when you are hoping to embark upon a lifestyle change of this nature. If you are feeling tired and sluggish and miserable, it is going to be highly unlikely for you to want to make the changes that need to be made, and especially difficult for them to stick when you do begin to make an effort. However, eating foods that are healthy for you and that help you to maintain your energy levels and your focus is a great way to embark upon a journey that will provide you with healing and improve your health.

In fact, in many cultures, food is considered to be a medicine. It is believed that if you eat well and the right foods at the right times of the day, you will be able to not only maintain a healthier body but also a better attitude and spirit all around. The ancient healing art of Ayurveda has been around for centuries and is still in use today because so many of the foods that are used as medicine have genuine anti-inflammatory and antibacterial properties that having them in your diet consistently can help you to prevent illness. There is actually some science to back that. If you eat properly, you are going to be able to provide your immune system with the resources that it needs in order to stave off infection and disease.

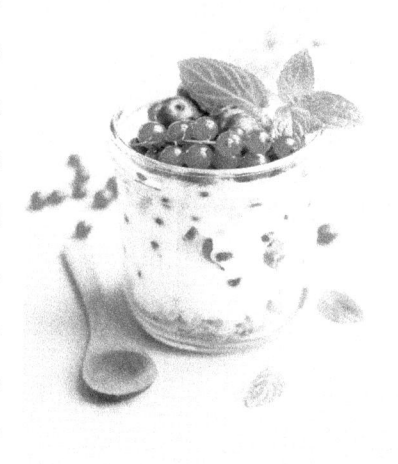

Unfortunately, the standard American diet too often lacks in fresh fruits and vegetables, even though it is common knowledge that they are jam packed with the vitamins and minerals that our bodies need to thrive. Without the proper types of food in our diets, it can be difficult to maintain high energy levels. At least when you are consuming a regular amount of fruits and vegetables, you can begin to notice a difference in your disposition.

You will also begin to notice a difference in your weight. If you are going from starchy and carb-filled foods to a diet higher in water-based foods that are full of fiber, your body will begin to eliminate the toxins that bind fat to them and allow you to begin a more rapid ascent into weight loss!

Chapter 8

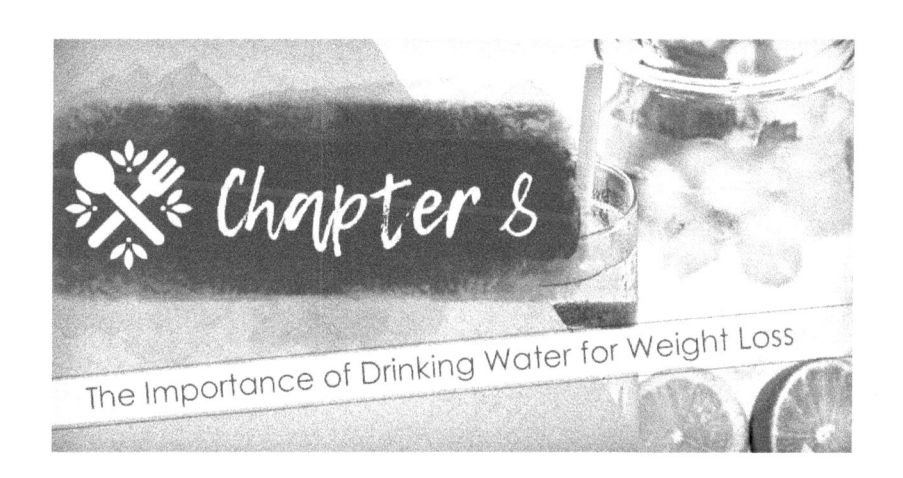

The Importance of Drinking Water for Weight Loss

Most people gain a lot of weight initially because it is very difficult to avoid drinks that are packed full of sugar. Many people's every day diets consist of soda or juice or smoothies, all of which contain higher than healthy levels of sugar. It is unhealthy for the body to be so consistently overloaded with sugars, and if this issue isn't addressed it can easily begin to pack on the pounds and make it difficult for your body to process the excessive sugars that it is consuming.

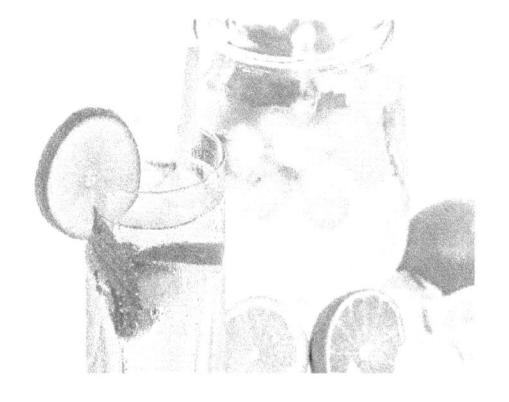

The importance of drinking water for weight loss is largely misunderstood. In fact, water in general is very underappreciated, especially in western culture where sugary and caffeinated drinks are far more coveted by the masses. These drinks are packed full of calories that can make it seem impossible to begin losing weight, no matter how much time and effort you put into it. Water is a low calorie alternative that is not only helpful in losing weight, but also beneficial in a whole plethora of other ways as well.

Water is hydrating and moisturizing, and can help clear up skin problems and provide our skin with a healthy glow. It can also contribute to having soft, well-hydrated skin that is pleasant to the touch. When we are able to provide our bodies with the proper amount of water, it can also help us to reduce headaches and to flush toxins from the body.

It can actually be very common for our bodies to confuse thirst signals with hunger signals. It is recommend that if you hear your stomach growling, that you begin to drink water first rather than eating. It can help you to begin to differentiate the feeling of hunger versus thirst. It can also help you to prevent consuming needless calories because you have mistaken your body's reaction to thirst for hunger. Always try to drink water when your stomach growls or you have hunger pangs, because the indication that you are thirsty is the same as when you are in need of food. A lot of people get confused by this, but it doesn't mean that you should eat every time that you think you are hungry. Just keep this in mind as a rule of thumb and you may be surprised by how easy it is to avoid consuming needless calories.

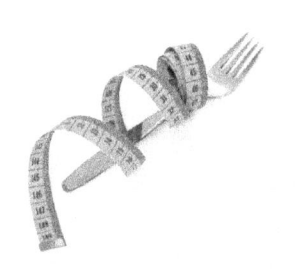

Something that not many people realize, is that water is an appetite suppressant. That means that, should you choose to drink an adequate amount of water, you will ultimately find that you are less hungry throughout the day. This may be especially true when you drink a glass of water before a meal. It will help you to suppress your appetite and keep it contained so that you aren't overeating during your meals.

It is an especially useful trick if portion control is a struggle that you are coping with. Drinking a glass of water before a meal can be one of the most beneficial and natural ways to prevent yourself from overeating that there is. It will also help your body in general to get a good amount of water so that you are able to focus. Much like getting enough fruits and vegetables, without an adequate amount of water in the diet, the human body tends to become sluggish and miserable. We are designed to run at our best on a good amount of water. It can be likened to the fuel that keeps our bodies moving at their greatest capacity.

The general amount of water that it takes to keep things moving smoothly is about 64 ounces daily. That will help you to have a decent grasp on your appetite and a sharper mental focus. When you are at your best mentally, it will help you to stay at your best physically as well. There will be a great amount of focus and perseverance required in achieving your goals, and if you are meeting you body's basic requirements then it will be a lot easier for you to do so.

Possibly the most incredible thing about drinking water is the fact that it can help you to boost your metabolism simply by drinking it. It gets your body primed to burn calories at an extended rate and allows the body to utilize your fat as fuel.

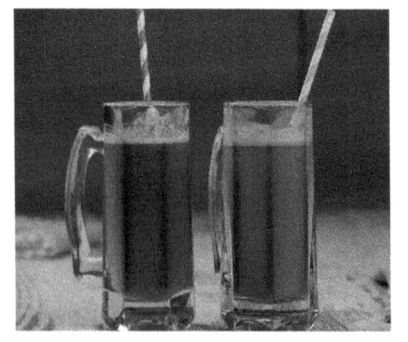

Another good reason that water aids in weight loss is that it helps to support the Overall, utilizing water as a way to lose weight is a great way to easily assist in a foolproof diet. It will be especially efficient if you are cutting out other types of drinks, particularly soda and other high-sugar juices and things like that. For the best results at weight loss you want to try to keep your sugar intake at a minimum, and replacing sugary drinks with water is a great way to begin to burn calories that are already there rather than putting more into your body.

If you find that drinking water and water alone is not working for you, perhaps because it is too plain, you could try tea or infuse your water with fruits or vegetables. Cucumber in particular makes a very refreshing way to infuse water and encourage you to drink more, presuming you like the taste of cucumber. If not, there are several other viable options that you could use, including but not limited to watermelon, lemon, or strawberries. These are all great and delicious ways to up your water intake without increasing the caloric content of your water by as large a percentile as you would were you to drink soda or juice.

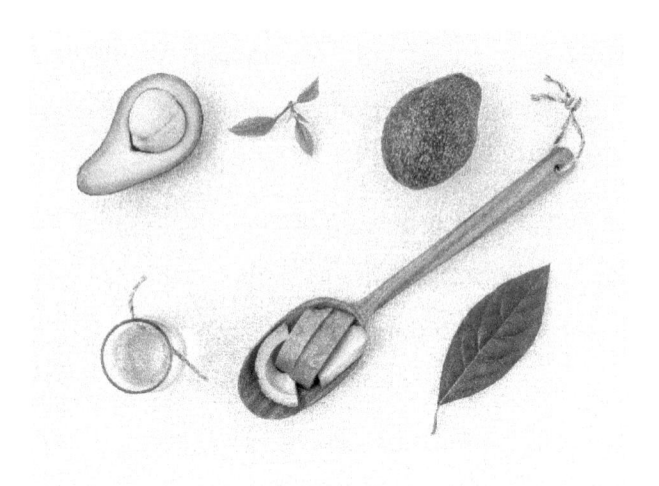

You may be wondering if juicing is a good idea, especially if you have seen all the documentaries and other research about juicing. The simple fact is that store bought juices contain concentrated amounts of sugars from the fruits contained within them and also added sugars from the process of creating a product that people will consume. It is not healthy. However, if you were to juice fruits and vegetables, that is a different story.

The catch here is that using a juicer to drink your fruits and vegetables rather than eating them will deplete the beverage from the healthy fibers that make fruits and vegetables so beneficial for the body. Rather than drinking pulp free juice, make sure to add in the fibers, at least a few, for best results. You should also avoid juicing a lot of fruits all at once, because you will simply be consuming what could essentially be considered as sugar water. Fruits are high in natural sugar, and if you are overloading your body with a juice that is primarily all fruit, it can be detrimental.

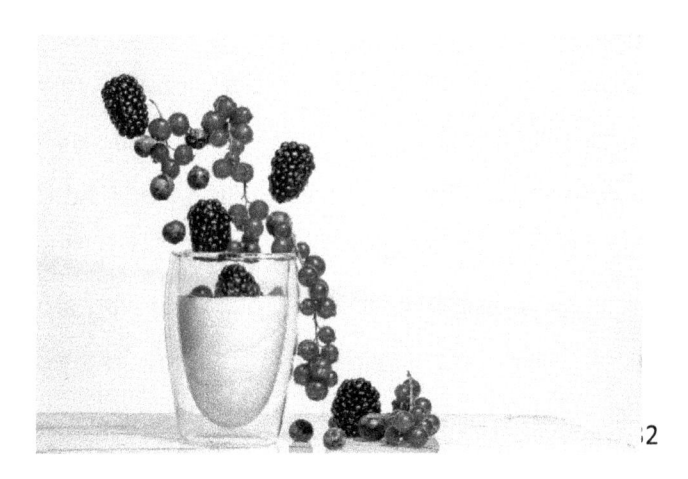

The trick here is to drink juices that are two parts vegetable and one part fruit, and add in some of the pulp so you are also getting the added benefit of the fibers that make fruits and vegetables extra healthy and good for weight loss. We will talk more about juicing in the last chapter, as there are many tips and tricks that can be utilized for weight loss. Especially if you are interested in a large variety of dietary options.

As a rule, consuming a good amount of water is the greatest thing you can do to boost your metabolism and jump start your ability to lose weight. Without a chance to rid the body of toxins and energize the cells, our bodies retain both water and fat and that can make it nearly impossible to achieve the bodies that we want to achieve. Accomplishing your goals can be easier than you think. Just make sure you are drinking approximately 64 ounces of water daily so that you are able to fully benefit from water intake in order to make your diet as foolproof as it can possibly be. You will be glad you did. It is such a simple and helpful tool in aiding in both weight loss and improving our overall health. Most people don't think twice about grabbing a soda over a water, but when you are making the time to think about what you are putting into your body before you do it, then you will do much better at losing weight over the long term! And that is the only foolproof way to truly make maintaining a healthy body into a lifestyle choice that you can stick with over the long haul.

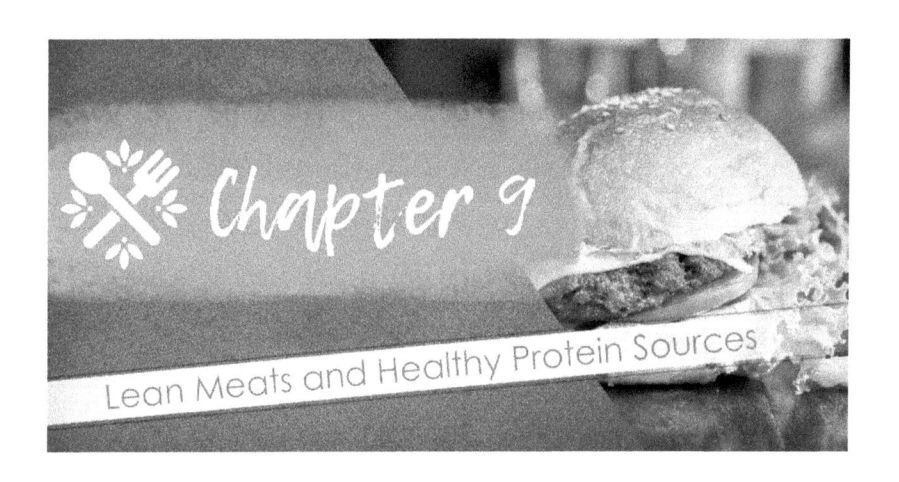

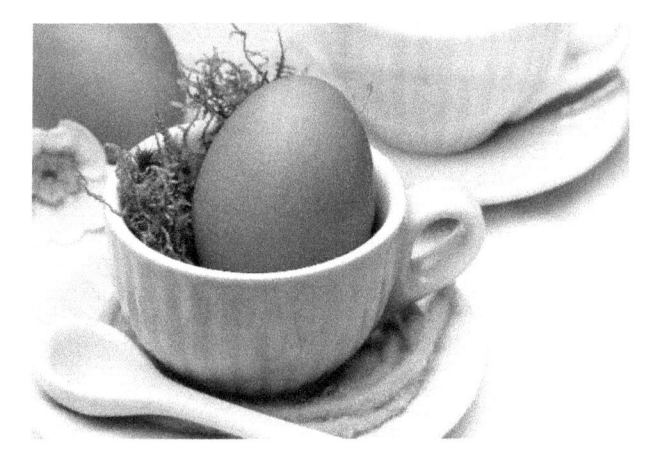

Chapter 9
Lean Meats and Healthy Protein Sources

One thing that has been proven time and again is that protein is great for the body for a variety of reasons. Not only does it help you to build muscle mass, but it also has a tendency to help to stave away hunger, which can be a great way to enforce portion control when it seems most impossible.

However, some protein sources are better than others, and if you want to make sure that you are encouraging your body to heal at the most rapid rate possible while building muscle that helps to burn fat quickly, you want to avoid protein sources that are actually going to be putting more fat into your body.

Lean protein sources are the best for you, especially if you want to lose weight effectively and do whatever it takes to maintain the lifestyle that you are creating for yourself. These sources of protein are important in your weight loss journey, and the following paragraph will outline the best lean protein sources that you can find, both animal based and plant or seed based.

Eggs are one of the best lean protein sources. They are filling and packed full of this particular nutrient. And you don't have to eat a whole lot of them to get a high amount of protein and a good boost of energy. This is a great snack to have post work out to help you to build muscle and burn fat all day long!

Lean meats are mostly poultry based, such as the white meat found in turkey or chicken. Red meats are more fatty and less lean, which can have an adverse effect on weight loss. Other lean protein sources include soy and seafood, though be careful about where you get your seafood from.

Unfortunately, some seafood is contaminated with pollutants such as mercury due to the coal factories so close to the oceans, and you also want to be wary of farmed fish as well. Look into ethically raised seafood if you are interested in adding that to your diet, and remember that making sound and informed choices about your food is the fastest way toward maintaining a foolproof diet for the rest of your life!

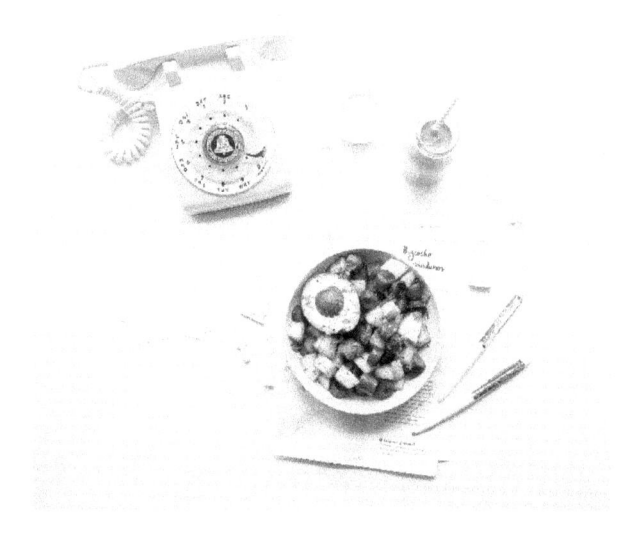

Other great lean protein sources include nuts and seeds, such as sunflower seeds, almonds, pistachios, cashews, walnuts, pumpkin seeds, and other commonly known seed and nut varieties that are packed with proteins and healthy fats.

Healthy fats are also important when it comes to weight loss. If you are eating unhealthy fats then you are bound to gain weight. However, healthy fats are essential to the body's makeup and can be very important to keep in the diet. They support your body and provide you with a great source of energy without making it excessively difficult to lose weight.

Healthy fats include things such as nuts and seeds, nut butters in particular, and also foods like avocado and olives. Even olive oil is a good source of healthy fat and can actually be beneficial for the body in the long term rather than detrimental. Fish is another source of healthy fat, so if you are able to find a good source of seafood, eating fish is a great way to keep the body lean and healthy without abandoning the hearty and savory meals that make your body and mind feel content.

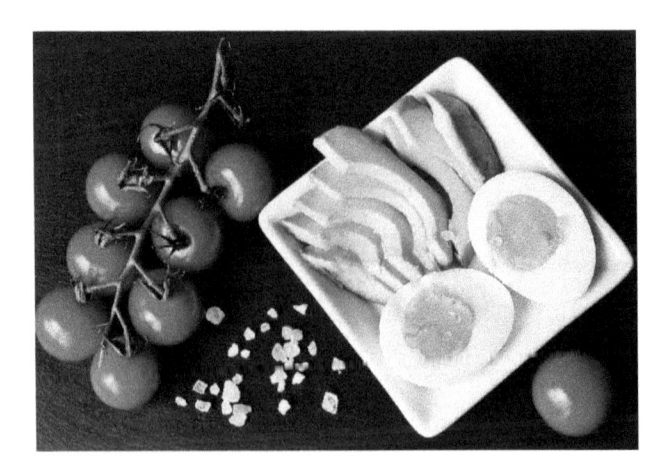

The difference between lean meat and fatty meat is often the source. All meat has at least a little bit of fat in it, but that is why it is so good for you to eat fish and other safe seafoods. These are full of healthy fat, not bad fat. Red meat in particular is higher in fat because the types of animals that they come from are bigger, stockier, and have a different type of diet than livestock that provides lean meat sources for consumption. Fish does not have saturated fats like the other types of meat, which makes it arguably the best choice for anyone who is going to be eating meat long term to sustain themselves and attempt to live as healthy a lifestyle as possible.

Overall, meat has good points and bad points, and if you are a vegan or vegetarian or simply just don't like a whole lot of meat, there are other protein options available. Remember, tofu is made of soy, as well as tempeh, and there are other types of foods that can provide you with good protein as well, such as nuts, nut butters, seeds, and even some leafy green vegetables!

Whatever your lifestyle choice happens to be, we can all eat great and make choices that will help us to be healthier and happier and more mentally alert than we ever have been before! It all starts with you. Educating yourself and starting in slow is the biggest key in creating a healthy lifestyle that will provide you with a foolproof way to lose weight and keep it off, starting now!

Chapter 10
Planning Meals and Other Tips and Tricks

Embarking upon any lifestyle change is going to take some organization. If you aren't fully prepared for it, it is bound to fail. What most diet plans don't talk about are the mental and emotional challenges that come with losing weight and making the changes that need made both mentally and physically before we are able to lose weight and keep it off.

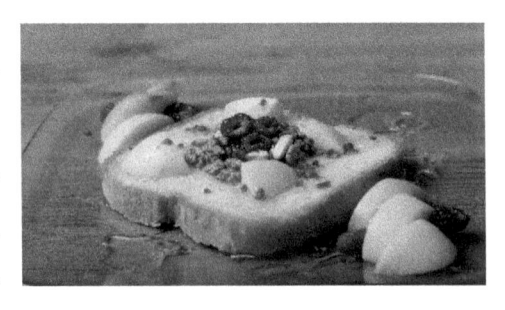

You have to be able to pinpoint the true source of your unhappiness before you will ever be able to address it. For example, if you are a compulsive over eater, why is that? Are you trying to fill an emotional void? If so, what left it there and how can you address it? Are you simply struggling with self-discipline? If so, why do you think that may be and what can you do to make yourself more reliable? Or is your issue more to do with the fact that you simply don't know a lot about cooking and find yourself falling back on the easiest possible options? Do you lack time and feel that cooking takes more than it is worth? If so, look into easy meal preparation guides and tips that will help you with making meals in the home in a way you are comfortable with and that will sustain you.

Paleo diet books are a great place to begin if you are a meat eater. The paleo diet tries to stay as close to a natural diet as possible and nourishes your body in a way that keeps out processed foods and the abundance of sugars present in them that make weight loss difficult.

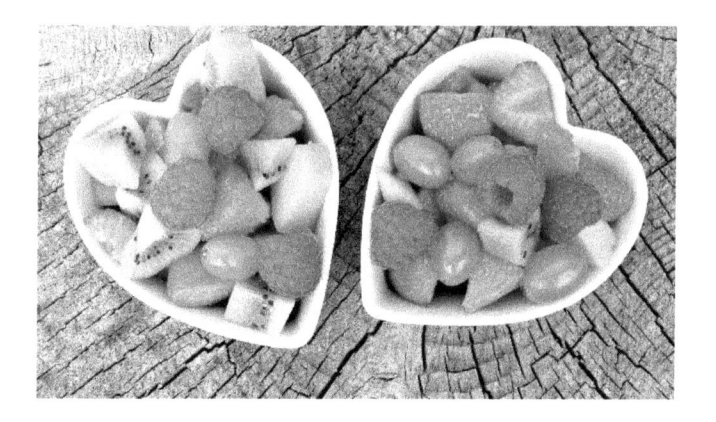

Juicing can be great, especially if you have a hard time eating fruits and vegetables in their natural forms. One great way to get yourself interested in juices is to add apples. Apples are good for you and have a natural but not overwhelming sweetness. As long as you are adding some of the natural fibers of the fruits and vegetables back into your juice, then adding an apple or two won't hurt a thing. In fact, it is a great way to get both nutrients and a delicious, sweet flavor into the juice you are drinking, whether it is full of vegetables you may not like or not!

If you don't mind drinking water and don't feel that juicing would be an essential way to get variety of drinks into your diet, then you should ignore this next tip. Most people I know struggle with drinking the right amount of water daily, and opt for more flavorful options. Spicing things up a little by adding variety in your water, and flavoring it with fruits and vegetables is one good way to get that variety.

Another trick you might want to employ is to make sure that you have drank at least half your necessary daily intake of water before indulging in other drinks that you find moderately healthy and more sugary or flavorful. Once you have had the proper amount of water in a day, you can reward yourself with something else that may be a little sweeter.

Although it is recommended to avoid all sugary and processed drinks in general in order to have the greatest effects, it is more important that you are living your life in a way that is bearable and manageable for you and you are making conscious choices in what you consume. Whether a diet succeeds or fails is often on your own shoulders; at least, the kind that attempts to change a lifestyle rather than looking for a quick fix to something that is not healthy to fix quickly.

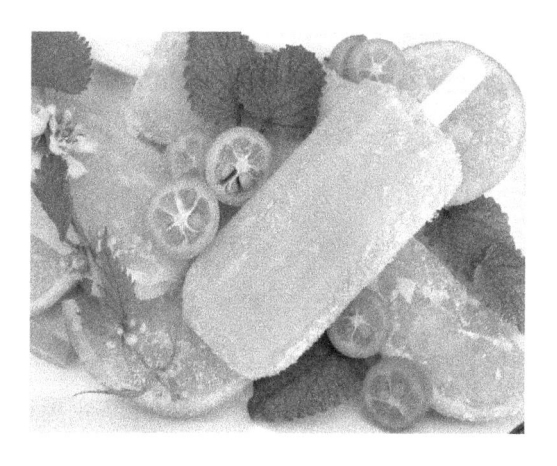

The real intention of the foolproof diet is to train yourself to have the willpower to make healthy choices that will change the way you view your dietary choices. If you feel that your choices are limited because you are not very creative in the kitchen with healthy foods, don't worry. You should see this as an opportunity to continue to learn and view each new experience in the kitchen as a chance to improve. Even if it starts out rocky, there are things that can make it easier.

For example, creating a meal plan is a great way to help you to get into the swing of things. There are many meal planners online that can help you to get the hang of getting an idea of what you are going to eat throughout the week. Stick with the foods outlined in this book. Lean meats and proteins, fruits, and vegetables. Eat starches in moderation, once or twice a week rather than daily as a staple. You will probably find it difficult at first, but they are full of sugars that make you even hungrier so you consume more food that ultimately breaks down into fat in your body. Drink at least 64 ounces of water daily, and avoid sugar and processed foods like the plague.

The paleo diet in general is a good guideline to follow; avoiding the unhealthy foods out there will really help you to stay balanced and provide you with a foolproof way to diet and create a lifestyle change that works best for you. One that is sure to last.

Conclusion

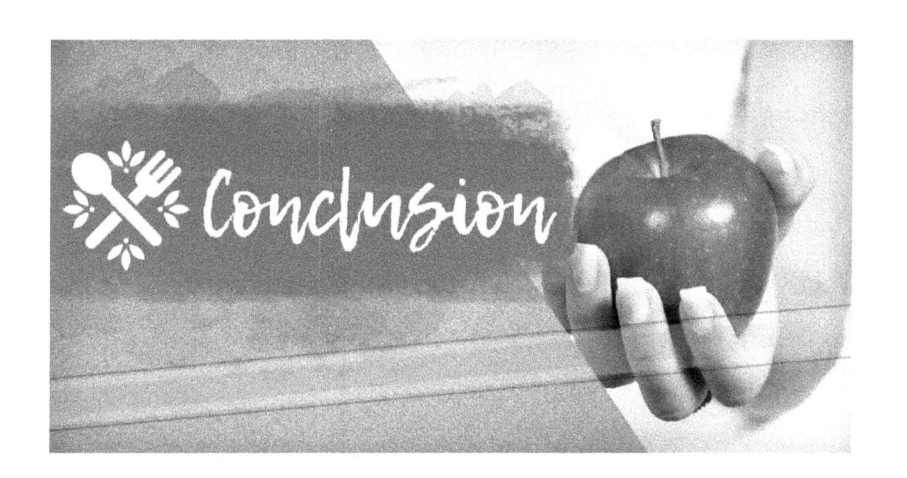

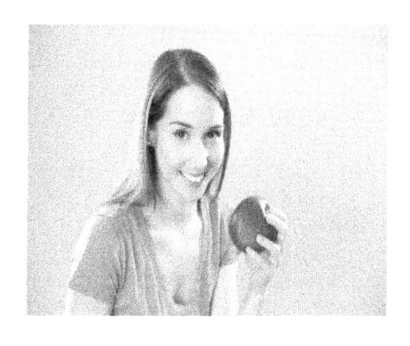

Everybody these days is looking for a foolproof diet; the best way to lose weight and keep it off. A fast, easy solution to the problems that have begun to plague us because we have gotten comfortable living an unhealthy lifestyle for far too long.

But what most fail to consider is the fact that it is our own minds, and our habits, that truly create the biggest boon. We rely on other people to try to help us dig ourselves out of a pit that only we have the tools to get out of. You are in control of your life. You will be the one responsible for making the choices that need to be made to change your lifestyle. And you are more than strong enough to do it.

Start out small. Take baby steps. Break your goals down into pieces that are manageable, and then begin to pursue your goals with confidence. Even if you relapse, even if you fall down, you have to have the courage and the confidence to get back up. It is up to you whether or not you succeed, and a foolproof diet is only going to be foolproof if you make it work for you and not the other way around.

What many people don't seem to understand is that you are important. You are valuable. We punish ourselves and make bad choices because we don't always value ourselves and lack the self love and discipline necessary in creating the life of our choosing. But all of that can end today, starting now. if you are willing to take an honest look at yourself and how you got to where you are now, you will have the resources at your disposal to make the changes you need made.

Rather than complicating your life with more and more and more fad diets and trends, what would really make a difference is in simplifying things down. Make simple food choices. Eat foods that are nourishing, healthy, and low in fat and sugar. Don't eat things that you already know are not good for you. It sounds simple, but unless you have addressed all the underlying issues that are causing you to have an issue with healthy eating, these simple rules of thumb will be harder and harder to abide by.

The foolproof diet begins and ends with you. All the diet books and advice in the world could tell you what to do, but at the end of the day it is up to you what you apply to your life. Following the guidelines that are present in the Foolproof Diet book will provide you with the tools you need in order to succeed and begin to live the life that you deserve, starting now!